Bad Breath Buster

Your Ultimate Resource for Eliminating Mouth Odor

Tracey J. Collins

Table Of Content

Introduction

Bad breath is a common and often embarrassing problem that affects many people. It can impact our personal and professional lives, affecting our confidence and self-esteem. There are many potential causes of bad breath, from poor oral hygiene to certain medical conditions, and the resulting odor can be difficult to eliminate.

This book, "Bad Breath Buster: Your Ultimate Resource for Eliminating Mouth Odor," is a comprehensive guide to understanding and treating bad breath. Whether you are struggling with chronic halitosis or simply want to improve your breath for social or professional situations, this book provides practical and effective solutions.

The Science of Bad Breath:
To effectively treat bad breath, it is important to understand the science behind it. In the first chapter of this book, we will explore the various causes of bad breath, including poor oral hygiene, diet, medical conditions, and lifestyle factors such as smoking. We will also discuss the biological mechanisms behind bad breath and how it affects our bodies.

Myths and Misconceptions:
There are many myths and misconceptions surrounding bad breath, which can make it difficult

to effectively treat. In the second chapter of this book, we will debunk common misconceptions about bad breath and provide accurate information to help you better understand the problem.

Oral Hygiene and Bad Breath:
Maintaining good oral hygiene is crucial for preventing and treating bad breath. In the third chapter of this book, we will provide practical tips and techniques for brushing, flossing, and using mouthwash to keep your mouth clean and fresh.

Natural Remedies:
While traditional oral hygiene practices are effective for preventing bad breath, there are also many natural remedies that can help freshen breath and improve overall oral health. In the fourth chapter of this book, we will explore natural remedies such as essential oils, herbs, and other home remedies that can be used to eliminate bad breath.

Over-the-Counter Solutions:
If natural remedies do not provide sufficient relief, there are many over-the-counter solutions available that can help eliminate bad breath. In the fifth chapter of this book, we will provide an overview of mouthwashes, sprays, and chewing gum that are designed to freshen your breath and improve oral health.

Prescription Medications and Bad Breath:

Certain prescription medications can also cause bad breath as a side effect. In the sixth chapter of this book, we will discuss medications that can cause bad breath and provide solutions for addressing the problem.

Bad Breath and Gum Disease:
Gum disease is a common condition that can contribute to bad breath. In the seventh chapter of this book, we will explore the link between gum disease and bad breath and provide strategies for preventing and treating gum disease.

Bad Breath and Dry Mouth:
Dry mouth, or xerostomia, is a condition in which the mouth does not produce enough saliva. This can lead to bad breath and other oral health problems. In the eighth chapter of this book, we will discuss the causes of dry mouth and provide strategies for preventing and treating the condition.

Bad Breath and Smoking:
Smoking is a major contributor to bad breath, as well as other oral health problems. In the ninth chapter of this book, we will explore the link between smoking and bad breath and provide strategies for quitting smoking.

Bad Breath and Medical Conditions:
Certain medical conditions can also contribute to bad breath, including sinus infections, acid reflux, and diabetes. In the tenth chapter of this book, we

will discuss these conditions and provide solutions for addressing bad breath as a symptom.

Managing Bad Breath in Social Situations:
Finally, in the eleventh chapter of this book, we will provide practical tips and tricks for managing bad breath in social and professional situations. Whether you are going on a first date or attending a job interview, this chapter will provide strategies for ensuring fresh breath and confident communication.

Conclusion:
"Bad Breath Buster: Your Ultimate Resource for Eliminating Mouth Odor" is a comprehensive guide to understanding and treating bad breath. By exploring the various causes of bad breath and providing practical solutions for prevention and treatment, this book aims to help readers achieve fresh breath and improved oral health.

Throughout the book, we have covered a wide range of topics, including the science of bad breath, myths and misconceptions, oral hygiene, natural remedies, over-the-counter solutions, prescription medications, gum disease, dry mouth, smoking, and medical conditions.

By reading this book, you will gain a thorough understanding of bad breath and the various factors that can contribute to it. You will also learn practical strategies for preventing and treating bad breath, as well as managing it in social situations.

Whether you are struggling with chronic halitosis or simply want to improve your breath for personal or professional reasons, "Bad Breath Buster" provides a wealth of information and guidance to help you achieve your goals.

So, what are you waiting for? Let's embark on this journey towards fresh breath and improved oral health!

Chapter 1

Understanding the Science of Bad Breath: The Causes and Mechanisms of Mouth Odor

Have you ever wondered why your breath sometimes smells bad, even when you brush and floss regularly? It turns out that there are a variety of factors that can contribute to bad breath, or halitosis, as it's medically known.

One of the primary causes of bad breath is the accumulation of bacteria in the mouth. The human mouth is home to millions of bacteria, which can feed on food particles and produce foul-smelling compounds like hydrogen sulfide and methyl mercaptan.

In addition to bacterial buildup, other factors can also contribute to bad breath. These include:

- Dry mouth: Saliva plays an important role in washing away bacteria and food particles in the mouth. When the mouth is dry, as can happen due to certain medications or medical conditions, bacteria can thrive and cause bad breath.

- Gum disease: Also known as periodontitis, gum disease is a common condition that can lead to bad breath. It occurs when the gums become inflamed and infected due to a buildup of plaque and tartar.

- Medical conditions: Certain medical conditions, such as diabetes, sinus infections, and liver or kidney disease, can cause bad breath.

- Foods and drinks: Certain foods and drinks, such as garlic, onions, and coffee, can leave a lingering odor in the mouth.

Now that we've explored the causes of bad breath, let's take a closer look at the mechanisms behind it.

As we mentioned earlier, bacteria in the mouth produce foul-smelling compounds as they feed on food particles. These compounds can also be produced when proteins in the mouth break down, a process known as proteolysis.

In addition to bacterial activity, other factors can also contribute to bad breath. For example, when we consume certain foods and drinks, like garlic and coffee, the compounds they contain can be absorbed into the bloodstream and carried to the lungs. From there, they can be exhaled and cause bad breath.

So, how can we prevent bad breath? The key is to maintain good oral hygiene habits, such as brushing and flossing regularly, using mouthwash, and cleaning the tongue. In addition, drinking plenty of water can help keep the mouth hydrated and prevent dry mouth.

In some cases, bad breath may be a symptom of an underlying medical condition, so it's important to see a healthcare provider if you're experiencing chronic halitosis.

Chapter 2

Myths and Misconceptions about Bad Breath: Separating Fact from Fiction

We'll be exploring some common myths and misconceptions about bad breath and separating fact from fiction in this chapter. Let's get started!

Myth #1: Bad breath is always caused by poor oral hygiene.

While it's true that poor oral hygiene can contribute to bad breath, it's not the only cause. As we discussed in the previous chapter, factors like dry mouth, gum disease, and medical conditions can also lead to bad breath. So, if you're brushing and flossing regularly and still experiencing bad breath, it's important to explore other potential causes.

Myth #2: Mouthwash can cure bad breath.

While mouthwash can help freshen breath in the short term, it's not a cure for bad breath. In fact, some types of mouthwash can actually contribute to dry mouth, which can make bad breath worse. It's important to use mouthwash as part of an overall oral hygiene routine, but it's not a substitute for regular brushing and flossing.

Myth #3: Minty gum or candy can cure bad breath.

While minty gum or candy can temporarily mask bad breath, they don't address the underlying causes. In fact, some types of gum or candy can actually contribute to bad breath by increasing saliva production and creating an environment where bacteria can thrive. Instead of relying on gum or candy, focus on maintaining good oral hygiene habits and exploring other potential causes of bad breath.

Myth #4: Bad breath is always noticeable.

While some cases of bad breath are quite noticeable, others may be more subtle. In fact, many people with chronic halitosis may not even be aware that they have bad breath. This is why it's important to maintain good oral hygiene habits and seek medical attention if you're experiencing chronic halitosis.

Myth #5: Bad breath is contagious.

Contrary to popular belief, bad breath is not contagious. While certain bacteria that contribute to bad breath can be transmitted through saliva, it's not possible to catch bad breath like you would a cold or the flu.

Now that we've separated fact from fiction when it comes to bad breath, let's explore some practical tips for preventing and treating it.

First and foremost, maintaining good oral hygiene habits is key. This includes brushing and flossing regularly, using mouthwash, and cleaning the tongue. Additionally, staying hydrated and avoiding foods and drinks that can contribute to bad breath, such as garlic and coffee, can help keep your breath fresh.

If you're experiencing chronic halitosis despite good oral hygiene habits, it's important to see a healthcare provider. They can help identify potential underlying causes and recommend appropriate treatments.

Chapter 3

The Link between Diet and Bad Breath: What You Eat Affects How Your Breath Smells

You may be surprised to learn that what you eat can have a big impact on how your breath smells. One of the primary ways that diet can impact bad breath is through the production of volatile sulfur compounds (VSCs).

VSCs are produced by the bacteria in our mouths when they break down certain types of food. This can lead to a foul-smelling odor that is often associated with bad breath.

So, what types of foods are most likely to cause bad breath? Here are a few culprits to watch out for:

1. Garlic and onions - These pungent foods are notorious for causing bad breath. This is because they contain sulfur compounds that are particularly potent when broken down by oral bacteria.

2. Dairy products - Milk, cheese, and other dairy products can contribute to bad breath in a couple of ways. First, they can cause a buildup of mucus in the

throat, which can lead to an unpleasant odor. Additionally, the proteins in dairy products can be broken down by oral bacteria, leading to the production of VSCs.

3.   Sugary foods and drinks - Sugar can feed the bacteria in our mouths, leading to an overgrowth that can contribute to bad breath. Additionally, sugary drinks like soda can contribute to dry mouth, which can exacerbate bad breath.

4.   Alcohol - Alcoholic beverages can contribute to bad breath in a couple of ways. First, they can lead to dehydration, which can make bad breath worse. Additionally, the breakdown of alcohol in the body can lead to the production of VSCs.

While it's important to be mindful of the types of foods and drinks you consume, it's also worth noting that some foods can actually help combat bad breath. Here are a few options to consider:

1. Fresh fruits and vegetables - These foods are high in water and fiber, which can help promote saliva production and flush out bacteria in the mouth.

2.   Green tea - Green tea contains compounds that can help kill the bacteria that contribute to bad breath.

3.   Probiotic foods - Probiotic foods like yogurt and kefir can help promote the growth of "good" bacteria in the gut and mouth, which can help combat bad breath.

In addition to being mindful of the types of foods you consume, it's also important to practice good oral hygiene habits. This includes brushing and flossing regularly, using mouthwash, and cleaning the tongue. If you're experiencing chronic halitosis despite these efforts, it's important to see a healthcare provider. They can help identify potential underlying causes and recommend appropriate treatments.

Chapter 4

Oral Hygiene and Bad Breath: Brushing, Flossing, and Mouthwash Techniques to Improve Breath Odor

It's no secret that proper oral hygiene is essential for maintaining fresh breath. In this chapter, we'll delve into some of the best practices for brushing, flossing, and using mouthwash to help eliminate bad breath.

First and foremost, let's discuss brushing. Brushing your teeth at least twice a day is a cornerstone of good oral hygiene. But it's not just about brushing frequently; it's also about brushing effectively. The American Dental Association (ADA) recommends using a soft-bristled brush and fluoride toothpaste. Be sure to brush all surfaces of your teeth, including the fronts, backs, and chewing surfaces. It's also important to brush your tongue to remove any bacteria that can contribute to bad breath. And don't forget to replace your toothbrush every three to four months or when the bristles become frayed.

Flossing is another crucial aspect of oral hygiene. Flossing helps remove food particles and bacteria from between teeth, where a toothbrush can't reach. The ADA recommends flossing at least once a day. To floss properly, use about 18 inches of floss and wrap it around your fingers, leaving about two inches between them. Use a gentle sawing motion to slide the floss between your teeth, being careful not to snap it against your gums.

Mouthwash can also be an effective tool for fighting bad breath. Mouthwash works by killing bacteria in the mouth, but it's important to note that it should never be a substitute for brushing and flossing. Look for mouthwashes that contain antibacterial agents such as chlorhexidine, cetylpyridinium chloride, or essential oils like thymol and eucalyptol. And when using mouthwash, be sure to swish it around in your mouth for at least 30 seconds before spitting it out.

In addition to these basic practices, there are other tips and techniques you can use to improve your oral hygiene and fight bad breath. Here are a few:

- Use a tongue scraper: As we mentioned earlier, bacteria can accumulate on the tongue and contribute to bad breath. A tongue scraper can help remove that bacteria and freshen your breath.

- Chew sugarless gum: Chewing gum can help stimulate saliva production, which can help wash away bacteria and food particles in the mouth. Just make sure to choose a sugarless gum to avoid adding more sugar to your diet.

- Drink plenty of water: Staying hydrated is important for many aspects of health, including oral health. Drinking plenty of water can help keep your mouth moist and rinse away bacteria.

- Avoid tobacco and alcohol: Both tobacco and alcohol can contribute to bad breath. Tobacco can dry out your mouth and leave an unpleasant smell, while alcohol can lead to dehydration and cause a similar effect.

By following these tips and techniques, you can improve your oral hygiene and reduce the likelihood of bad breath. And if you're still experiencing persistent bad breath despite these efforts, it may be time to see a dentist or doctor to rule out any underlying medical conditions.

Chapter 5

Natural Remedies for Bad Breath: Essential Oils, Herbs, and Other Home Remedies to Try

If you've tried all the usual methods to combat bad breath, from brushing and flossing to using mouthwash, but still can't seem to shake the odor, it might be time to try some natural remedies. There are many essential oils, herbs, and other natural remedies that can help freshen your breath and improve your oral hygiene. In this chapter, we will explore some of the best natural remedies for bad breath.

One of the most effective natural remedies for bad breath is essential oils. Peppermint oil, for example, has a fresh and invigorating scent that can help mask bad breath. You can use it by adding a few drops to your toothpaste, mouthwash, or even directly to your tongue. Other essential oils that are good for bad breath include tea tree oil, lemon oil, and eucalyptus oil.

Herbs are another great way to freshen your breath naturally. Parsley, for example, is a natural breath freshener that contains chlorophyll, a natural deodorizer. Chewing on fresh parsley leaves after a meal can help neutralize bad breath. Mint is another herb that can help freshen your breath, and it can also stimulate the production of saliva, which helps wash away food particles and bacteria that cause bad breath.

You can also use natural home remedies to freshen your breath. One popular remedy is apple cider vinegar. Simply dilute a tablespoon of apple cider vinegar in a glass of water and use it as a mouthwash. This can help neutralize the pH of your mouth and kill bacteria that cause bad breath. Another effective home remedy is baking soda. Mix a teaspoon of baking soda in a glass of water and use it as a mouthwash to help neutralize acids in your mouth and kill odor-causing bacteria.

In addition to these remedies, there are also several foods that can help improve your breath. One of the most well-known is yogurt, which contains healthy bacteria that can help combat the bacteria that cause bad breath. Crunchy fruits and vegetables, such as apples and carrots, can also help scrub your teeth and freshen your breath.

While these natural remedies can be effective in combating bad breath, it's important to remember that they are not a substitute for good oral hygiene habits. Brushing and flossing regularly, as well as visiting your dentist for regular check-ups and cleanings, are still the best ways to maintain good oral health and prevent bad breath.

In summary, natural remedies such as essential oils, herbs, and home remedies can be effective in combating bad breath. However, they should be used in conjunction with good oral hygiene habits, such as brushing, flossing, and regular dental check-ups. So, if you're looking for a natural way to freshen your breath, try incorporating some of these remedies into your oral hygiene routine and see if they make a difference!

Chapter 6

Over-the-Counter Solutions for Bad Breath: An Overview of Mouthwashes, Sprays, and Chewing Gum

Bad breath is a common problem that affects people of all ages. While practicing good oral hygiene and maintaining a healthy diet can go a long way in preventing bad breath, sometimes these measures may not be enough. In such cases, over-the-counter solutions can be an effective way to freshen your breath and combat mouth odor. In this chapter, we will explore some of the most popular over-the-counter solutions for bad breath.

Mouthwashes are a popular solution for bad breath. They work by killing the bacteria that cause bad breath, as well as freshening the breath with a pleasant taste or scent. There are many different types of mouthwashes available on the market, including those that contain alcohol and those that are alcohol-free. While alcohol-based mouthwashes can be effective in killing bacteria, they may also cause dry mouth, which can actually exacerbate bad breath. For this reason, many people prefer to use alcohol-free mouthwashes. Some of the key ingredients to look for in a mouthwash include cetylpyridinium chloride, chlorhexidine, and hydrogen peroxide, all of which have been shown to be effective in killing bacteria and freshening breath.

Another popular over-the-counter solution for bad breath is chewing gum. Chewing gum stimulates the production of saliva, which can help to wash away bacteria and food particles that can cause bad breath. Additionally, many chewing gums are flavored with mint or other pleasant scents, which can mask bad breath and freshen the breath. However, it is important to choose sugar-free chewing gum, as sugar can actually contribute to bad breath.

In addition to mouthwashes and chewing gum, there are also sprays that can be used to freshen your breath. Breath sprays work by delivering a burst of pleasant scent or flavor into the mouth, which can help to mask bad breath. Some breath sprays also contain antibacterial ingredients, which can help to kill the bacteria that cause bad breath. When choosing a breath spray, it is important to look for one that is sugar-free and alcohol-free, as these ingredients can actually make bad breath worse.

Finally, there are also oral care products that are specifically designed to combat bad breath. For example, tongue scrapers can be used to remove bacteria and food particles from the tongue, which is a common source of bad breath. Additionally, there are toothpaste and gels that are formulated to combat bad breath, such as those that contain zinc or chlorine dioxide. These products work by neutralizing the sulfur compounds that cause bad breath, leaving the mouth feeling fresh and clean.

While over-the-counter solutions can be an effective way to combat bad breath, it is important to remember that they are not a substitute for good oral hygiene and a healthy diet. Additionally, if your bad breath is persistent or severe, it may be a sign of an underlying medical condition, and you should consult with a healthcare professional to determine the underlying cause of your bad breath.

In conclusion, over-the-counter solutions for bad breath can be an effective way to freshen breath and combat mouth odor. Mouthwashes, chewing gum, sprays, and oral care products can all be useful in combating bad breath, but it is important to choose products that are sugar-free and alcohol-free and to remember that they are not a substitute for good oral hygiene and a healthy diet.

Chapter 7

Prescription Medications and Bad Breath: How Certain Drugs Can Cause Mouth Odor and What to Do About It

Many prescription medications can cause bad breath, also known as halitosis. In this chapter, we will discuss the most common medications that can lead to mouth odor and what you can do to manage it.

Firstly, it is essential to understand why some medications cause bad breath. Some medications can cause dry mouth or xerostomia, a condition where the mouth produces less saliva than usual. Saliva plays a crucial role in washing away bacteria and food particles that can cause bad breath. When there is not enough saliva, bacteria can accumulate in the mouth, leading to an unpleasant odor.

Some medications that can cause dry mouth and bad breath include:

- Antidepressants: Many types of antidepressant medications can cause dry mouth and related bad breath, including selective serotonin reuptake inhibitors (SSRIs), tricyclic antidepressants, and monoamine oxidase inhibitors (MAOIs).

- Antihistamines: These medications, often used to treat allergies or cold symptoms, can also lead to dry mouth and bad breath.
- Blood pressure medications: Certain types of blood pressure medications, such as diuretics and beta blockers, can cause dry mouth and bad breath as a side effect.
- Anti-anxiety medications: Benzodiazepines, often used to treat anxiety disorders, can also contribute to dry mouth and bad breath.
  And others like; Pain medications, Diuretics, Antipsychotics, Muscle relaxants, Chemotherapy drugs, etc.

If you are taking any of these medications and notice that your breath smells unpleasant, talk to your doctor. They may adjust your medication or prescribe an additional medication to help manage the side effects.

There are also some things you can do to manage dry mouth and bad breath while taking medication. Drinking plenty of water can help keep your mouth hydrated and wash away bacteria. Chewing sugar-free gum or sucking on sugar-free candy can stimulate saliva production and help keep your mouth moist.

Another way to manage bad breath caused by dry mouth is to use a moisturizing mouthwash. There are many over-the-counter types of mouthwash designed to help relieve dry mouth and freshen breath. Look for a mouthwash that contains fluoride to help protect your teeth from decay.

It is also important to practice good oral hygiene habits while taking medication. Brush your teeth twice a day with fluoride toothpaste and floss daily to remove any food particles and bacteria that can cause bad breath.

If you are experiencing bad breath despite practicing good oral hygiene and managing dry mouth, it may be a sign of an underlying medical condition. In some cases, bad breath can be a symptom of an infection, such as gum disease or a respiratory infection. Talk to your doctor or dentist if you have persistent bad breath or other symptoms, such as bleeding gums or a persistent cough.

In summary, certain prescription medications can cause dry mouth and bad breath. If you are experiencing mouth odor while taking medication, talk to your doctor about adjusting your medication or prescribing additional medication to manage side effects. Drinking plenty of water, chewing sugar-free gum, and using moisturizing mouthwash can also help manage dry mouth and bad breath. Finally, practicing good oral hygiene habits and seeking medical attention if symptoms persist is essential to maintaining good oral health.

Chapter 8

Bad Breath and Gum Disease: How Gum Disease Affects Your Breath and What You Can Do About It

When we talk about bad breath, we usually think of it as a problem that originates in the mouth. However, bad breath can also be a symptom of gum disease, a condition that affects the gums and supporting tissues of the teeth. Gum disease is a common problem, affecting millions of people worldwide. In fact, it is one of the leading causes of tooth loss in adults.

What is gum disease?

Gum disease, also known as periodontal disease, is an infection of the gums and supporting tissues of the teeth. It is caused by the buildup of plaque, a sticky film of bacteria that forms on the teeth. If plaque is not removed through regular brushing and flossing, it can harden into tartar, which can only be removed by a dental professional.

The early stage of gum disease is called gingivitis, which is characterized by red, swollen, and bleeding gums. If left untreated, gingivitis can progress to periodontitis, which can lead to tooth loss and other serious health problems.

How does gum disease cause bad breath?

One of the most common symptoms of gum disease is bad breath. This is because the bacteria that cause gum disease produce volatile sulfur compounds (VSCs), which have a foul odor. These VSCs can be detected on the breath and can make it smell unpleasant.

In addition to causing bad breath, gum disease can also lead to other oral health problems that can contribute to bad breath. For example, gum disease can cause the gums to recede, which can expose the roots of the teeth. This can create pockets between the teeth and gums where bacteria can grow and produce VSCs.

Gum disease can also cause tooth decay and cavities, which can also contribute to bad breath. When bacteria in the mouth feed on sugars and starches, they produce acid that can erode the enamel of the teeth, leading to cavities and decay.

What can you do to prevent gum disease and bad breath?

The best way to prevent gum disease and bad breath is to practice good oral hygiene. This includes:

- Brushing your teeth twice a day with a fluoride toothpaste.

- Flossing at least once a day to remove plaque and food particles from between your teeth.
- Using an antiseptic mouthwash to kill bacteria and freshen your breath.
- Visiting your dentist regularly for check-ups and professional cleanings.

In addition to good oral hygiene, there are other steps you can take to prevent gum disease and bad breath. These include:

- Eating a healthy diet that is rich in fruits, vegetables, and whole grains.
- Avoiding sugary and starchy foods that can feed the bacteria that cause gum disease and bad breath.
- Quitting smoking, which can increase your risk of gum disease and other oral health problems.
- Managing any underlying health conditions that can contribute to gum disease, such as diabetes.

If you have gum disease, your dentist may recommend a deep cleaning procedure called scaling and root planning. This involves removing plaque and tartar from the teeth and smoothing the roots of the teeth to help the gums reattach to the teeth.

In some cases, your dentist may also recommend medication or surgery to treat gum disease. However, these treatments are usually reserved for more advanced cases of gum disease and should be discussed with your dentist.

Conclusion

Bad breath can be embarrassing and frustrating, but it is a problem that can be treated. If you have bad breath, it may be a symptom of gum disease. By practicing good oral hygiene and taking steps to prevent gum disease, you can improve your oral health and keep your breath smelling fresh. If you're struggling with persistent bad breath, don't hesitate to talk to your dentist or healthcare provider for guidance and treatment options. With the right approach, you can conquer bad breath and enjoy a happier, healthier life.

Chapter 9

Bad Breath and Dry Mouth: Causes, Consequences, and Treatment Options

Bad breath can be caused by a variety of factors, including poor oral hygiene, gum disease, certain medications, and even some medical conditions. One often-overlooked cause of bad breath is dry mouth, also known as xerostomia. In this chapter, we'll explore the link between bad breath and dry mouth and discuss some treatment options to alleviate this issue.

First, let's talk about what dry mouth is and what causes it. Dry mouth occurs when there isn't enough saliva in the mouth. Saliva helps to wash away food particles and bacteria that can lead to bad breath. When there's not enough saliva, bacteria can accumulate in the mouth, leading to a buildup of odor-causing compounds.

There are many possible causes of dry mouth, including certain medications, medical conditions, and lifestyle factors. Some medications, such as antihistamines, antidepressants, and diuretics, can cause dry mouth as a side effect. Medical conditions such as Sjogren's syndrome, diabetes, and Parkinson's disease can also cause dry mouth. Smoking and drinking alcohol can also contribute to dry mouth.

So, how does a dry mouth lead to bad breath? When there's not enough saliva in the mouth, bacteria can grow and multiply more easily. As bacteria break down food particles, they release odor-causing compounds such as volatile sulfur compounds (VSCs). These compounds are responsible for the unpleasant odor we associate with bad breath.

If you have a dry mouth, there are several things you can do to help alleviate the problem. One of the simplest things you can do is to drink more water. Staying hydrated can help to keep your mouth moist and wash away bacteria and food particles. Chewing sugar-free gum can also help to stimulate saliva production.

There are also a number of over-the-counter products that can help to alleviate dry mouth. Mouthwashes and sprays specifically designed for dry mouth can help to moisturize the mouth and freshen breath. Some products contain xylitol, a natural sweetener that can help to stimulate saliva production. You can also try using a humidifier in your home to keep the air moist.

If dry mouth is caused by a medication you're taking, talk to your doctor about alternatives. They may be able to switch you to a different medication that doesn't cause dry mouth as a side effect. If you have a medical condition that's causing dry mouth, treating the underlying condition can often help to alleviate the dryness and bad breath.

In conclusion, dry mouth can be a major contributor to bad breath. If you're experiencing dry mouth, there are a variety of treatment options available to help alleviate the problem. Drinking more water, chewing sugar-free gum, and using over-the-counter products designed for dry mouth can all help to stimulate saliva production and freshen breath. If your dry mouth is caused by a medication or medical condition, talk to your doctor about alternative treatments. By addressing the underlying cause of dry mouth, you can help to eliminate bad breath and enjoy a healthier, more comfortable mouth.

Chapter 10

Bad Breath and Smoking: How Tobacco Use Affects Breath Odor and Strategies for Quitting

We all know that smoking is bad for our health, but did you know that it can also have a significant impact on your breath? That's right, smoking can cause bad breath, and it's not just because of the smell of smoke on your clothes and hair. In this chapter, we'll explore how smoking affects your breath odor and provide strategies for quitting.

How Smoking Causes Bad Breath

Smoking causes bad breath in a number of ways. First, tobacco smoke contains more than 4,000 chemicals, many of which are toxic and can lead to oral health problems such as gum disease and tooth decay. These oral health issues can contribute to bad breath. In addition, smoking can dry out your mouth, which can also cause bad breath. Saliva is essential for washing away food particles and bacteria in your mouth, and when your mouth is dry, those particles and bacteria can accumulate and cause a foul odor.

Smoking can also affect your taste buds, making it more difficult to taste and smell food properly. This can lead to a decreased sense of taste and smell,

which can make it harder to detect bad breath.
Finally, smoking can lead to an increased
production of mucus, which can further contribute
to bad breath.

Strategies for Quitting Smoking

Quitting smoking is not easy, but it is one of the best
things you can do for your overall health, including
your oral health and breath odor. Here are some
strategies to consider:

1. Talk to your doctor: Your doctor can provide
   resources and support to help you quit
   smoking. They may recommend nicotine
   replacement therapy, prescription
   medications, or counseling.

2. Set a quit date: Choose a date to quit smoking
   and stick to it. Make a plan for how you will deal
   with cravings and triggers.

3. Use distractions: Find activities to keep your
   hands and mind busy, such as knitting or crossword
   puzzles, when you feel the urge to smoke.

4. Seek support: Join a support group or talk to
   friends and family about your decision to quit.
   Having a support system can make a big difference.

5.   Practice good oral hygiene: While quitting smoking, it's important to maintain good oral hygiene to help combat bad breath. Brush and floss regularly and consider using mouthwash to freshen your breath.

6.   Use sugar-free gum or mints: Chewing sugar-free gum or sucking on sugar-free mints can help combat the dry mouth and bad breath associated with smoking.

7.   Stay motivated: Remember why you want to quit smoking and focus on the benefits, such as better breath, improved health, and saving money.

In conclusion, smoking can cause bad breath in a number of ways, including contributing to oral health issues and dry mouth. Quitting smoking can be a challenge, but it's worth it for the positive impact it can have on your overall health, including your breath odor. By using these strategies, you can successfully quit smoking and improve your breath odor at the same time.

Chapter 11

Bad Breath and Medical Conditions: How Certain Health Problems Can Cause Mouth Odor and How to Address Them

Bad breath, or halitosis, is a common condition that affects people of all ages and backgrounds. While it's not always a simple case of brushing and flossing when it comes to bad breath. Sometimes, the cause of your mouth odor can be rooted in a medical condition. In this chapter, we'll explore some of the health problems that can lead to bad breath and what you can do to address them.

Sinus Infections and Post-Nasal Drip

If you suffer from chronic sinusitis or allergies, you may be familiar with the unpleasant odor that accompanies these conditions. Sinus infections can cause mucus buildup in the sinuses, leading to post-nasal drip and a persistent bad taste in your mouth. The bacteria that thrive in this environment can produce an odor that is often described as "rotten eggs."

If you suspect that a sinus infection or post-nasal drip is the culprit behind your bad breath, it's important to address the underlying condition. See a doctor to determine the best course of treatment, which may include antibiotics, decongestants, or allergy medication.

Gastrointestinal Issues

Believe it or not, your digestive system can play a role in your breath odor. Gastrointestinal problems such as acid reflux, GERD, and ulcerative colitis can cause stomach acids and food particles to back up into your mouth, resulting in bad breath.

If you suspect that a gastrointestinal issue is causing your bad breath, make an appointment with a gastroenterologist. They can perform tests to determine the root cause of your symptoms and recommend appropriate treatment options.

Dry Mouth

We touched on the topic of dry mouth in Chapter 9, but it's worth mentioning again here. A dry mouth can be caused by a number of factors, including certain medications, dehydration, and medical conditions such as Sjogren's syndrome. When your mouth doesn't produce enough saliva, bacteria can thrive and cause bad breath.

If you suffer from dry mouth, there are several steps you can take to address the problem. Stay hydrated by drinking plenty of water, chew sugar-free gum to stimulate saliva production, and talk to your doctor about adjusting your medication if dry mouth is a side effect.

Diabetes

People with diabetes are at a higher risk for developing gum disease, which, as we discussed in Chapter 8, can cause bad breath. In addition, high blood sugar levels can lead to a fruity or sweet odor on the breath, known as "ketone breath."

If you have diabetes and are experiencing bad breath, it's important to keep your blood sugar levels under control. This may involve adjusting your diet, taking medication, and working closely with your healthcare team to manage your condition.

Liver and Kidney Disease

Liver and kidney disease can also cause bad breath. In liver disease, a buildup of toxins in the body can lead to a foul odor in the breath. Kidney disease can cause a metallic taste in the mouth, as well as bad breath due to high levels of urea in the bloodstream.

If you suspect that liver or kidney disease is causing your bad breath, see a doctor immediately. These conditions can be serious and require prompt medical attention.

In conclusion, bad breath can be a sign of an underlying medical condition. If you're experiencing persistent mouth odor despite practicing good oral hygiene, it's important to see a doctor to rule out any underlying health problems. With the right treatment and management, you can improve your breath and maintain optimal overall health.

Chapter 12

Managing Bad Breath in Social Situations: Tips and Tricks for Managing Your Breath When You're Out and About

Bad breath can be a real nuisance, especially when you're out in public. Whether you're on a date, at a business meeting, or simply hanging out with friends, having bad breath can make you feel self-conscious and embarrassed. Fortunately, there are plenty of things you can do to manage bad breath in social situations. In this chapter, we'll go over some tips and tricks for managing your breath when you're out and about.

1. Carry Breath Mints or Gum
   One of the easiest ways to manage bad breath on the go is to carry breath mints or gum with you. Not only do these items freshen your breath, but they also stimulate saliva production, which helps to wash away bacteria and food particles that can cause bad breath. Look for sugar-free options to avoid adding unnecessary sugar to your diet.

2. Drink Water

Drinking water is another simple way to manage bad breath on the go. Not only does it help to rinse away bacteria and food particles, but it also keeps your mouth hydrated, which helps to prevent dry mouth. A dry mouth can lead to bad breath because saliva helps to neutralize the acids that can cause bad breath.

3.   Avoid Certain Foods
Certain foods, such as garlic, onions, and spicy foods, are notorious for causing bad breath. If you know you'll be in a social situation where bad breath is a concern, it's best to avoid these foods altogether. Opt for foods that are less likely to cause bad breath, such as fruits and vegetables.

4.   Practice Good Oral Hygiene
Practicing good oral hygiene is crucial when it comes to managing bad breath, especially when you're out and about. Be sure to brush your teeth twice a day and floss daily to remove any food particles and bacteria that can cause bad breath. You can also use a tongue scraper to remove any bacteria that may be lurking on your tongue.

5.   Try a Breath Freshening Spray

Breath freshening sprays are a convenient way to freshen your breath when you're on the go. These sprays work by neutralizing the bacteria that cause bad breath and leaving your mouth feeling clean and refreshed. Keep a small bottle in your purse or pocket for easy access.

6. Chew on Parsley
    Believe it or not, chewing on a sprig of parsley can help to freshen your breath. Parsley contains chlorophyll, which is a natural deodorizer that can neutralize bad breath. Keep a small bag of parsley in your purse or pocket and chew on a sprig whenever you need to freshen your breath.

7. Avoid Smoking and Drinking Alcohol
    Smoking and drinking alcohol can both lead to bad breath, so it's best to avoid these activities when possible. If you do smoke or drink alcohol, be sure to rinse your mouth out with water or use a breath freshening spray afterward.

8. Keep Your Mouth Moist
    As we mentioned earlier, dry mouth can lead to bad breath. To keep your mouth moist, try sipping on water throughout the day or sucking on sugar-free candy or mints. You can

also try using a saliva substitute, which is a
product that helps to replace the saliva that
your body isn't producing.

9. Practice Mindful Breathing
Believe it or not, the way you breathe can
affect your breath odor. When you breathe
through your mouth, you're more likely to
have bad breath because it dries out your
mouth and allows bacteria to thrive. Practice
mindful breathing by breathing through your
nose and taking slow, deep breaths. This will
help to keep your mouth moist and prevent
bad breath.

10. Visit Your Dentist Regularly
Regular dental check-ups and cleanings are an
essential part of managing bad breath. Your
dentist can check for signs of gum disease,
tooth decay, and other oral health issues that
can cause bad breath. They can also remove
any built-up plaque and tartar that may be
contributing to your mouth odor.

During your dental appointment, make sure to
discuss any concerns you have about your
breath. Your dentist can provide advice on
how to improve your oral hygiene routine or
recommend specific treatments, such as

antimicrobial mouthwashes or prescription
toothpaste.

11. Stay Hydrated
Dehydration can contribute to bad breath, as
it leads to a dry mouth where bacteria can
thrive. To combat this, make sure to drink
plenty of water throughout the day. This can
help keep your mouth moist and wash away
food particles and bacteria that can cause
odor.

In addition to water, you can also try drinking
green tea. Green tea contains polyphenols,
which are natural compounds that can help
reduce the growth of bacteria in the mouth.

12. Try Sugar-Free Gum or Mints
Sugar-free gum or mints can be a quick and
easy way to freshen your breath on the go.
Chewing gum stimulates saliva production,
which can help wash away bacteria and
neutralize odors. Mints can also help mask
bad breath temporarily.

However, it's important to choose sugar-free
options, as sugary gum or mints can actually
contribute to bad breath by feeding the
bacteria that cause it.

13.   Address Underlying Health Issues
If you have chronic bad breath that doesn't improve with lifestyle changes or over-the-counter remedies, it may be a sign of an underlying health issue. Certain medical conditions, such as respiratory infections, diabetes, and liver or kidney disease, can cause bad breath.

If you suspect that an underlying health issue is causing your bad breath, it's important to consult with your healthcare provider for a proper diagnosis and treatment plan.

14.   Don't Ignore Persistent Bad Breath
While occasional bad breath is common, persistent bad breath that doesn't improve with self-care measures may be a sign of a more serious underlying issue. It's important to take persistent bad breaths seriously and seek professional help if needed.

In conclusion, bad breath can be an embarrassing and frustrating issue to deal with, but there are many ways to address it. By practicing good oral hygiene, staying hydrated, and addressing any underlying health issues, you can improve your breath odor and feel more confident in social situations. Don't be afraid to talk to your healthcare

provider or dentist if you need help managing your
bad breath.